How to Stop Alcohol Craving

Lucinda Robinson

HOW TO STOP ALCOHOL CRAVING

Dr. Hulda Clark has discovered in her research the true cause and cure for alcohol craving. It is NOT a social disease. It is NOT a character defect. It is NOT an acquired habit. It is a combination of a chemical pollutant and mold that occupy the pleasure producing part of the brain that causes the craving for alcohol. This chemical and mold can be passed to a child while in the mother's womb. Using an all natural supplement regimen, the desire for alcohol and all its deadly side effects can be permanently eliminated in a few days. This has helped many, many people become permanently alcohol free using these discoveries.

Dr. Clark found the element beryllium usually is eliminated by the liver, but when the liver is disabled or over taxed, the chemical circulates freely in the bloodstream. She found that the chemical beryllium (found in coal products, coal oil, gasoline, kerosene, hurricane lamp oil, hurricane lamps, antique lamps, paint solvents, automotive products, paint cleaners, solvent cleaners, cigarette lighters, dry cleaning fumes, etc.) circulates in the bloodstream and lands at the addiction center of the brain (this center produces the pleasure sensing chemicals). This chemical is very reactive with alcohol. The two together in the brain cause certain neurotransmitters in the brain to be released that should not be released and restrict the release of neurotransmitters that should be released. This brings on the high or the depression of the alcoholic condition.

She also found that a mold common in food and alcoholic beverages (ergot mold) works with alcohol at the addiction center to make each other more toxic and reactive.

The pleasure producing part of the brain is usually carefully controlled by other chemicals so that not too much pleasure or happiness can be experienced. The site where the offending beryllium can land is normally the site for glutamate. When glutamate can not land there, the joy and happiness center cannot function, producing low level chronic depression and the craving for a time out of the depression, which translates into a craving for alcohol. The more beryllium present, the worse the depression. Supplementing the diet with glutamine (which the body turns into glutamate) helps boot out the beryllium. (It has been found that at least 3 grams of glutamine should be taken daily by those with depression and alcohol craving.)

When alcohol is put on the skin (tinctures, lotions, aftershaves, colognes, gasoline, petroleum solvents, etc.), inhaled (perfumes), or put in the mouth (mouthwashes, OTC medicines, alcoholic beverages, etc.) or produced in the intestines by fermentation (as by Candida yeast), a substance named salsol is formed. Salsol reacts very quickly with beryllium. At the pleasure producing site, the two together produce large quantities of pleasure producing chemicals. This is the alcoholic "high". You can feel this alcoholic "high" without ever drinking an alcoholic beverage if you have a Candida yeast infection in your intestines!!

As the beryllium is removed by natural means (by glutamine and by thioctic acid [otherwise known as alpha lipoic acid]), the salsol also disappears.

In order to eliminate the depressions in between alcoholic highs, to regulate the normal sense of well being and happiness without alcoholic consumption, and to eliminate the craving for alcohol, two things have to be avoided and eliminated from the body- beryllium and ergot mold. 10 grams (or 10,000 mgs. of Vitamin C- ester, buffered) in 3 divided doses daily will destroy the ergot. Taking at least 3 grams of glutamine daily and 600 mgs. alpha lipoic acid daily will remove the beryllium and salsol. An high B-complex tablet (B-75 or B-100) and 500 mgs. niacin amide taken 3 times a day will help the neurotransmitters to recover quickly. A GOOD, COMPREHENSIVE MULTI-VITAMIN AND MULTI-MINERAL SUPPLEMENT IS ALSO RECOMMENDED TO HELP FILL IN ALL NUTRITIONAL DEFICIENCIES CAUSED BY ALCOHOL CONSUMPTION. Green Vibrance is one such formula.

If you have no ergot or beryllium, and yet force yourself to consume alcohol, you will still have impaired brain and neurological responses from the alcohol alone. But the constant craving will not be there, if the ergot and beryllium are eliminated. This is another and different problem that should be dealt with. Some people drink alcohol just for the lightheaded, reality subduing feeling, not to fulfill a craving. But if alcohol is consumed regularly even for THIS reason, there is still much brain and liver damage, as well as multiple nutritional deficiencies created. IF YOU HAVE PROBLEMS YOU NEED TO DEAL WITH, GET HELP FROM A CHRISTIAN COUNSELOR. If there is some reality you are trying to escape, get away from the source, if possible. If you are constantly receiving negative messages from someone close to you, remove yourself from their presence. If you are tired, get more rest. If you tire too quickly on your job you must work, find out the foods and supplements that will increase your stamina and sense of well being. If there is no joy in your life except what is brought on by an alcohol high, you need spiritual peace with God and constant joy will be a by-product.

Even though a person who craves alcohol may stop drinking alcohol by sheer will power, the offending chemicals will stay in the brain unless removed by this method. If the offending chemicals are not removed, the craving will remain for YEARS. I personally had an uncle who was an alcoholic, but joined AA. He told me YEARS after he totally quit drinking that every moment of every day he craved alcohol, but by sheer personal will power he decided he would never drink again because of the great suffering he caused every one around him when he was drunk. During this time of abstinence, HE HAND DUG AN IN-GROUND SWIMMING POOL FOR HIS FAMILY and HAND BUILT AND PERSONALLY MANAGED A FAMILY RESTAURANT just to keep himself busy and off alcohol. How I wish he knew this information before he died that Dr. Clark has recently discovered!!

To insure the beryllium does not come in contact with you, there are several precautions you can take. Remove all hurricane or antique lamps from the home. Washing does not remove the chemical. Remove all stored paints, thinners, solvents, lighters including barbecue lighters from the home. They can be stored in an out building NOT attached to the home. Switch to all electric heating. The garage door should be permanently sealed off from the rest of the house or the garage itself should be closed and never used again to store the car, lawnmower, small engine lawn or garden tools or machines, or chemicals mentioned above. People with alcoholic cravings should never work as a painter, near or with automotive products, or in a dry cleaning business (independent painters have the highest percentage of alcoholism of any profession!!!) The pathways in the brain opened and maintained by the beryllium will be filled quickly again, even after the beryllium is removed, if the beryllium is ever present in the future.

How is it that some people can have a drink and not even think about alcohol for months and others think about it constantly and must have it on a daily basis? The answer has been found. Only those who have the beryllium and ergot are "addicted". Although taking in alcohol at anytime is not health building for anyone, the person who can just have one glass of wine and never care if he has another alcoholic drink again or not does not have the ergot/beryllium problem-THAT IS WHY THEY CAN TAKE OR LEAVE ALCOHOL. It is only when the ergot/beryllium is present that the craving is there.

FACTS ABOUT ALCOHOL

Every single time you consume alcohol, you kill off some brain cells.

Red wine keeps down blood fats, but so does red grape juice (and purple and white grape juice, also).

THERE IS ABSOLUTE PROOF THAT DRINKING ALCOHOL WHILE PREGNANT CAN PERMANENTLY DAMAGE YOUR UNBORN CHILD!

Beer contains brewer's yeast, a substance very high in energy producing B-complex vitamins. If the diet is very low in B-complex vitamins because few whole grains or greens are eaten or if the diet is very high in fats or sugars, there will be a craving for B-complex vitamins. Some people get their only and greatest dose of these from beer. Therefore, they associate a calming of the nerves and energy boost from the B-complex vitamins in beer while getting a very dangerous dose each of alcohol and ergot at the same time. They would be much better off taking a high potency B-complex tablet (B-75 or B-100) with every meal and leaving the mold and alcohol laced beer alone.

Even small amounts of alcohol affect the liver, brain, pancreas, duodenum, and central nervous system for the worse. It suppresses the immune system and affects the metabolic chemical reactions IN EVERY SINGLE CELL IN THE BODY. Daily consumption of alcohol shortens the life 10 to 15 years or more.

The liver can regenerate cells if part of the liver is removed, but if the cells are damaged by alcohol consumption, those cells can not reproduce.

Alcoholics have a much higher rate of mouth, throat, stomach, liver, colon, and breast cancer. They also have higher blood pressure, lower testosterone levels (decreased sex drive), higher blood vessel dilation (rosy skin), higher rates of congestive heart failure, more miscarriages, and more birth defects in their children than can be found in the non-drinking population.

If you can not go 24 hours without craving alcohol or thinking about it constantly, or looking forward to the next time you can get an alcoholic drink, you have an alcohol craving caused by the above factors. You are only free of it if not having another drink would never bother you at all. Buy the non-harmful supplements listed here and start on the road to being craving free and much healthier. If you are diligent in taking the supplements, you will start not craving the alcohol in a very short time- in a few days or in 2 or 3 weeks.

HOW TO GET THE ENERGY OF AN ALCOHOLIC HIGH WITHOUT ALCOHOL

When your energy sags, drink 100% orange juice, 100% blue grape juice, fresh carrot juice, or fresh parsley juice. These give you instant and long term energy and build up your health at the same time. Drinking these several times a day will keep blood sugar levels constant. Using these is much more effective than taking in carbonated, sugar-laden, caffeine loaded soft drinks AND their effects last much longer AND there are no bad side effects from them.

Raw sunflower seeds have every nutrient known to man except Vitamin C. If your energy is dropping, eat these to provide everything your body needs to get going strong again.

People who are under stress or who work long, hard hours can use B-complex vitamins (B-75 or B-100) many times a day to keep their energy levels up with no harmful side effects. If you take in too much, you just eliminate the excess through the urine. Take one tablet 3 to 8 times a day, as needed.

RELIEF FOR THE ADDICTION

For those of you who have fought for great periods of time against the craving, the time for remorse, guilt, sorrow, regret, hopelessness, self conflict, and compromised consciences is over. The problem is purely chemical and can be corrected in a relatively short period of time.

PATIENT SCHEDULE

LUCINDA ROBINSON
NATURAL HERBAL THERAPY
815A WYNNSHIRE DRIVE
HICKORY, NC 28601 USA
www.naturalherbaltherapy.info
naturalherbaltherapy@gmail.com
PH# 828-358-0609

PATIENT NAME:

DATE:

PRODUCT	WHEN ARISING	BREAKFAST	10:00 AM	LUNCH	3:00 PM	DINNER	BEFORE SLEEP
ESTER,BUFFERED VIT. C		3,000 MGS.		3,000 MGS.		4,000 MGS.	
GLUTAMINE		1500 MGS.				1500 MGS.	
ALPHA LIPOIC ACID		300 MGS.				300 MGS.	
NIACIN AMIDE		500 MGS.		500 MGS.		500 MGS.	
B-100 COMPLEX TABLET		1		1		1	

About the author-

Lucinda Robinson is an herbalist since 1973 from Hickory, North Carolina, USA. She is a Messianic/Nazarene Israelite believer. She was called by Yah in 1967 and gave her life to Him in faith and obedience in June of 1970. She is married to David and has 8 grown children and 8 grandchildren. She attended Cornell University where she studied child development, nutrition, consumer advocacy, and communications. She home birthed 7 of her children and homeschooled all 8 children for a total 14 years. She loves to study nutrition, herbal and natural cures for disease, the use of essential oils for healing, the history of the paganization and heathenization of the church, the true role of women from a Scriptural perspective, home industries, Scriptural archeology, the 4,000 plus year history of Messianic Judaism, the history of dress and dress design, organic gardening, and vegan cooking and raw food preparation.

Lucinda helps individuals in their homes or care facility to address their chronic and critical health needs as a natural health care worker as well as gives lectures, seminars, and has a video course for herbal cure enthusiasts.

She also travels as natural medical missionary, helping people with their health. and holds "health parties".

She counsels by appointment at her office and by phone, Skype audio and video, e-mail, and regular mail. You may contact her by e-mail at naturalherbaltherapy@gmail.com, by phone or Skype video at 1-828-358-0609, or by mail at 815 A Wynnshire Drive, Hickory, North Carolina, USA 28601.

Lucinda Robinson is not medical doctor and has never claimed to be a medical doctor. Every client asking for help comes with a medical doctor's diagnosis in hand before counseling can start. Lucinda does not diagnose or distribute any herbal supplements. She is an herbalist counseling clients about the well known, publicly published, and proven natural treatments that have proven over many years to be effective for certain health problems using herbs, vitamins, minerals, enzymes, probiotics, and other non-invasive physical treatments. Lucinda takes no responsibility for any effects that may come from anyone trying her suggested treatments and their results in that particular person. There are so many variable possibilities that affect health that an absolute certain outcome can not be guaranteed, especially if they are not under Natural Herbal Therapy's counseling's direct contact and supervision.

www.ingramcontent.com/pod-product-compliance
Lightning Source LLC
Chambersburg PA
CBHW070747310526
45791CB00028B/1675